# EXERCISES FOR
# CANCER WELLNESS

## William Smith

### with Contributions by Jo Brielyn

### Foreword by Kenneth Adler, M.D.

 **hatherleigh**

# ))) hatherleigh

Hatherleigh Press is committed to preserving and protecting the natural resources of the earth. Environmentally responsible and sustainable practices are embraced within the company's mission statement.

Visit us at www.hatherleighpress.com and register online for free offers, discounts, special events, and more.

*Exercises for Cancer Wellness*
Text copyright © 2015 William Smith

Library of Congress Cataloging-in-Publication Data is available.
ISBN: 978-1-57826-571-8

Cover Design by Heather Daugherty
Interior Design by Nick Macagnone
Photography by Catarina Astrom

Printed in the United States
10 9 8 7 6 5 4 3 2 1

**Disclaimer**
Consult your physician before beginning any exercise program. The author and publisher of this book and workout disclaim any liability, personal or professional, resulting from the misapplication of any of the following procedures described in this publication.

# Table of Contents

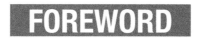

# FOREWORD

## by Kenneth Adler, M.D.

When I first started caring for people with cancer 35 years ago, I watched as my patients suffered from side effects of surgery, radiation, and chemotherapy treatments that were often as devastating as the disease itself. Treatments led to severe deconditioning. Drugs caused muscle weakness, severe fatigue, neuropathy, and weight gain; a patient's basic metabolism could be severely altered. And there was little we physicians could do to ease our patients' suffering. Our standard advice at the time was to suggest they get rest and avoid physical activity.

Today we know better. We tell them to get up and exercise. According to the National Comprehensive Cancer Network, moderate aerobic exercise such as riding an exercise bike or taking a brisk walk can significantly reduce cancer fatigue, and enhance one's sense of well-being. One recent study indicated that physical activity after a breast cancer diagnosis may be beneficial in improving quality of life, reducing fatigue, and assisting with energy balance. It may even lead to improved survival rates, but additional research is needed to confirm this. Two other recent studies (both focusing on colon cancer patients) have shown that higher levels of physical activity post-diagnosis may reduce the risk of cancer recurrence and increase survival rates.

Regular exercise can also help people undergoing cancer treatment to control their weight as another unhappy side effect of many oncology drugs is that they can stimulate appetite and lead to substantial weight gain.

Fortunately, exercise programs for cancer patients are now more readily available than ever. Many hospitals offer a full complement of exercise and wellness programs. More and more community centers, gyms, and yoga studios are developing fitness classes for cancer patients. Many of my own patients in New Jersey have enrolled in our local Livestrong program at the YMCA, which has given them a renewed sense of physical well-being after treatment. I've been thrilled to see some of my patients train to such a level that they've competed in 10K races, marathons, and even triathlons.

In their thoughtfully structured, expertly written *Exercises for Cancer Wellness,* William Smith and his collaborator Jo Brielyn address the fundamental importance of fitness during and after cancer treatment. A trainer, rehabilitation specialist, and triathlete, Mr. Smith puts forth in the book an exercise roadmap that will enable cancer patients to better navigate the road to wellness and recovery. He writes in a way that offers a clear, accessible understanding of how cancer and its treatment affects the body, and then explains exactly what patients can do to mitigate the impact of their illness and reconnect with their often depleted physical selves.

As I see it, *Exercises for Cancer Wellness* stands as evidence of how far cancer care has come since the 1970s, when all we had to offer our patients was a prescription to "stay off your feet." As a hematologist-oncologist, my goal for all of my patients has always been to help them attain the best possible quality of life. I look forward to recommending this excellent guide to help get them there.

—Kenneth Adler, M.D.,F.A.C.P.
Carol Simon Cancer Center at Morristown Medical Center, Regional Cancer Care Associates

# CHAPTER ONE

# A New Approach to Cancer Wellness

Whether you or a loved one have recently been diagnosed with cancer, or are currently at some point in treatment or recovery, you are already aware that cancer changes your life and the lives of those around you. And, while it is important for everyone to make healthy lifestyle decisions—like eating a nutritiously balanced diet and participating in physical activity on a regular basis—it is even more imperative for cancer patients and survivors to make smart decisions in regards to their health.

Implementing healthy lifestyle habits will help build a stronger, healthier you, better suited to combat the symptoms and side effects associated with cancer and its treatments. Making positive life changes during and after cancer treatment may also lessen the risks of a recurrence or relapse, as well as lower the chances of developing a second cancer. Cancer patients and survivors are also more likely to develop other chronic health issues (such as diabetes, heart problems, obesity, high blood pressure, and high cholesterol). Building and maintaining healthy lifestyle practices and habits can help to reduce the risks of those issues occurring.

The information provided in this chapter is intended to help you cope with some of the issues that occur among individuals living with cancer. The following sections will provide practical lifestyle tips for improved health for cancer patients and survivors.

## Defining Cancer

Cancer is not simply one disease. Rather, cancer can be considered as being many diseases categorized together. There are over 100 different types of cancer, and they can begin in almost any part of the body. The term **cancer** refers to diseases characterized by the growth of abnormal cells in the body that divide without control and have the potential to invade and destroy other normal tissues. These cells often form masses called **tumors**, although some forms of cancer (like leukemias and many types of lymphomas) do not form solid tumors.

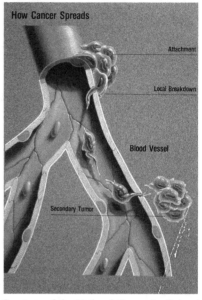

Courtesy of the National Cancer Institute at the National Institutes of Health.

Tumors present as either benign or malignant:

**Benign tumors** are not cancerous. Cells in benign tumors do not spread to other areas of the body. Benign tumors can often be removed, and usually do not reappear.

**Malignant tumors** are cancerous. Cells in malignant tumors can attack nearby tissues and spread to other areas of the body. When cancer spreads from one part of the body to another, it is called **metastasis.**

Most cancers are named for the organ or type of cell in which they first appear. Cancer cells may sometimes enter the lymph nodes or the bloodstream and spread to other parts of the body. When this process (metastasis) occurs, the cancer is still named for the area where it started. For instance, if breast cancer progresses into the lungs, it is referred to as *metastatic* breast cancer, not lung cancer

## Common Classifications of Cancer

The following are the most common areas where cancer can originate, named after their point of origin:

- **Carcinomas:** Cancers that start in the skin or in the tissue on the surface of internal glands and organs are named carcinomas. Included in this group are breast cancer, lung cancer, prostate cancer, and colorectal cancer.

- **Lymphomas:** Lymphomas are cancers that begin in the lymphatic system, which is the body's network of glands and vessels that work to fight infection. This group includes Hodgkin lymphoma and non-Hodgkin lymphoma.

- **Sarcomas:** Cancers that originate in connective tissues are considered sarcomas. Connective tissue includes fat, blood vessels, muscles, bones, nerves, cartilage, and deep skin tissues. Examples of sarcoma cancers are osteosarcoma or osteogenic sarcoma (cancer in the bones), fibrosarcoma (cancer in the fibrous tissue), and angiosarcoma (cancer of the blood vessels).

- **Leukemias:** Leukemias are cancers that start in the blood-forming tissues—such as bone marrow and the spleen. Among the cancers classified as leukemias are acute myeloid leukemia, chronic myeloid leukemia, acute lymphocytic leukemia, and chronic lymphocytic leukemia.

Of course, since there is such a variety of cancer types and unique situations, not all cancer patients will experience the same symptoms and side effects.

The following are some of the most common symptoms and side effects cancer patients can experience, along with practical tips for improving one's health, for individuals living with cancer.

## Fatigue

The majority of people with cancer experience a noticeable difference in energy level. During treatment with radiation and chemotherapy, fatigue is a common complaint. But fatigue is an experience that goes beyond simply feeling tired. It is a tiredness in the body and the brain, one that does not seem to improve even after rest. Fatigue can become severe and limit the individual's level of activity, as well as their desire to be active. This inactivity can in turn lead to loss of muscle function, so it is important to remain active.

Tips to avoid fatigue include:
- Plan your daily routine for activity around the times when you feel the best. Be sure to include active hobbies that you enjoy.
- Research shows that regular aerobic exercise will, in fact, help reduce fatigue, so make that a priority.
- Spend time outdoors. The fresh air will invigorate your senses, and the change in scenery will help break up the monotony and improve your mood.
- Eat a nutritious, balanced diet that includes protein—like meat, eggs, milk, and legumes—unless your physician has placed you on a diet that restricts these items.
- Pay attention to your fluid intake. Generally, it is advised to drink about 8–10 glasses of water each day.
- Avoid caffeine, alcohol, chocolate, and nicotine in the evening.
- Try to keep a smart balance of activity and rest throughout the day, one that does not interfere with your nighttime sleeping habits. If you must nap, limit it to under 30 minutes, and then do something active soon after waking.
- Remember that it is acceptable to ask for help from loved ones when you need it.

## Anxiety and Stress

It is normal to feel a great number of conflicting emotions when dealing with any serious disease. Cancer patients may find their feelings run the entire emotional gamut, with fear, stress, and anxiety often topping the list. It is important to find productive, effective ways to manage and work through these feelings in order to allow you to cope more effectively. Stress and anxiety can compound other symptoms such as fatigue, constipation, and diarrhea, as well as disturbances with sleeping and eating. It may also promote further or more frequent abuse of smoking tobacco, alcohol, and illicit drugs.

Tips to avoid stress and anxiety include:

- Practice breathing exercises and relaxation techniques to help control stress and anxiety.
- Make time for regular practice of physical activity and hobbies.
- Talk to your doctor or nurse about your feelings and the amount of stress in your life. For example, let them know if fear is keeping you from making decisions about your treatment, or if you are having conflict in your relationships.

## A Simple Breathing Exercise

Practicing a simple breathing exercise throughout the day will help relax your body, calm and refocus your thoughts, decrease fatigue, and increase oxygenated blood flow (which can decrease pain).

Learning how to focus and control your breath is one of the fundamental steps in meditation and relaxation. Close your eyes and take normal, deep breaths. Pay attention to how the air flows in through your nose and out of your mouth. Store the breath in your stomach, not the chest, in between inhales and exhales.

When you take slow, deep inhales through the nose, focus on how your lower chest and abdomen fill with air like a balloon. Hold that air in for five seconds, then slowly exhale, allowing the abdomen and chest to slowly deflate. Continue this practice of deliberate breathing for at least five minutes each day.

## A Quick Stress and Anxiety Relieving Exercise

Sometimes, moments of stress or anxiety may creep into your day. Try this quick, natural way to help "take a breather" and regain focus and energy.

Take a deep breath. Let it out naturally, and then try to push out a little more air. By practicing this regularly, you will build up the muscles between your ribs. Before long, you'll find yourself exhaling deeper and longer.

Over time, this conscious exhalation technique will become a healthy, unconscious habit you practice when you feel stressed or anxious.

## Deep Breathing

This breathing exercise sounds so simple that it almost seems unnecessary. However, once you start actually practicing deep breathing, you will wonder why you haven't been breathing like that all along! Deep breathing is much more effective for your body and mind than the shallow breaths people grow accustomed to taking throughout the day. This simple technique is an ideal form of relaxation before you go to bed.

Take a slow, deep breath in through the nose. Allow the breath to slowly and fully escape out of your mouth. Continue this technique and you will feel your heart rate slow and your mind and body relax.

## Loss of Appetite and Nausea/Vomiting

Many people who have cancer, especially those currently going through radiation and chemotherapy, experience issues with loss of appetite, nausea, vomiting, or some combination of these symptoms. Yet maintaining healthy nutrition is particularly necessary while receiving cancer treatment. Proper nutrition aids the body in healing, fighting infection, and preserving overall health. Cancer (and the treatments for cancer) can affect your body in different ways, sometimes changing the way foods taste, how you swallow or chew your food, or what foods your body can tolerate.

Tips to avoid loss of appetite, nausea, and vomiting include:
- Keep a log of the times when you feel nauseous to help determine what is making you sick.
- Stick to small, frequent meals instead of three large meals each day.
- Always have grab-and-go foods available, both at home and when you're out, especially items like dry crackers (which will help settle an uneasy stomach).
- If food odors are affecting your appetite, try eating foods with a pungent smell (like broccoli) while they are lukewarm or cold.
- Drink liquids between meals, instead of with your food.
- Participate in light exercise to help stimulate your appetite.
- If you are experiencing nausea, consider avoiding your favorite foods for a while—if you attempt to eat them and get nauseous, you may associate that food with getting sick.

- Avoid wearing tight-fitting clothes. These may add to your stomach discomfort.
- Stay away from eating fatty, greasy fried foods.
- Rinse your mouth with water, lemonade, or ginger ale to decrease bitter tastes.
- Remember that tart foods or drinks can often help settle an upset stomach.
- Experiment with different foods and seasonings to find ones that you can tolerate.
- Speak to your physician about anti-nausea medications or appetite stimulants if you are unable to eat or keep food down.

## Constipation

Constipation is a common complaint amongst cancer patients. Constipation refers to a condition where a person is unable to empty his or her bowels. It happens when the body absorbs more water than normal, or when food is moving more slowly through the bowel system. Common factors that contribute to the development of constipation are diet, inadequate fluid intake, a lack of exercise, medication side effects, and bowel obstructions. However, it can also be a presenting symptom of cancer. It may occur later, as a side effect of a growing tumor or cancer treatment. Constipation can cause other discomforts such as pain and cramping, swelling in the abdomen, nausea and vomiting, appetite loss, and the inability to urinate.

Tips to avoid constipation include:
- Increase your daily intake of fiber. Note that if you have adhesions or tumors that narrow your bowel, your doctor may suggest a low-fiber diet (or low-residue diet) instead; the narrower areas may block and cause fiber to back up in the bowel.
- Drink more liquids, including warm beverages, to help get the bowels moving.
- Engage in light exercise (which may also help stimulate your appetite).
- Talk to your physician about whether or not stool softeners will be beneficial for you.

## Diarrhea

Diarrhea is a physical issue that involves the person having frequent, loose, or watery bowel movements. Diarrhea may be caused by cancer, chemotherapy, and radiation therapy; however, it may also be due to conditions completely unrelated to cancer (like food intolerances). Make sure that you consult with your physician to narrow down the cause of your diarrhea.

Tips to avoid diarrhea include:
- Increase the amount of fluids you are drinking to avoid dehydration.
- Limit caffeine, alcohol, lactose products (dairy), orange juice, prune juice, spicy foods, and foods that are high in fat or fiber.
- Consume small, frequent meals instead of larger ones.
- Eat foods that are easier for your stomach to tolerate and digest, like the BRAT diet. The BRAT diet consists of bland and binding foods—Bananas, Rice, Applesauce, and Toast—and is frequently recommended for individuals recovering from diarrhea or an upset stomach.
- Increase your sodium and potassium sources to help replace nutrients your body loses due to diarrhea.

## Mouth and Throat Issues

Proper care for the mouth and throat is important for individuals with cancer. Cancer patients often experience sores, irritation, bleeding, and dryness (which are associated with some of the chemotherapy drugs used to treat the disease). Mouth sores can also become painful and infected, so it is wise to practice good oral hygiene.

Tips to avoid mouth and throat irritation include:
- Avoid tart, spicy, or acidic foods that will further irritate sores and other issues in the mouth and throat.
- Stay away from eating rough, coarse foods that may irritate the mouth and throat.
- Try eating food with sauce or gravy to make them easier to swallow.
- Use a straw for drinks or soups.
- Eat food when it is lukewarm instead of extremely hot or cold.
- Puree foods in a blender before consuming them.
- Drink liquids frequently to keep your mouth moist.
- Suck on hard candy or popsicles to help with a dry mouth.

## Hair Loss

The majority of cancer patients who undergo chemotherapy *will* lose their hair. Hair loss may happen anywhere on the body: the head, the face, limbs, or pubic area are some common areas. The drugs used in chemotherapy target rapidly-growing cells in the body. They are unable to distinguish between cancer cells and other fast-growing cells in the body, like hair follicles. Whether or not hair loss occurs is dependent on the type and dosage of the chemotherapy drug. Normally, hair loss starts 1–3 weeks after treatment begins. Hair typically grows back after treatment is finished, but some individuals may notice hair reappearing while they are still receiving chemotherapy treatment. The regrowth period for hair varies greatly, taking anywhere from 3–12 months.

Tips for dealing with cancer-related hair loss include:
• Consider cutting your hair short or shaving your head when hair loss begins to speed up the process.
• Clean and moisturize your scalp often to prevent skin problems.
• Avoid using blow dryers, curling irons, and other heat-styling appliances when your hair is thinning.
• Use mild shampoos and soft hair brushes.
• Wear sunscreen, hats, wigs, or other head coverings to protect your scalp from the sun.
• Choose fun, colorful accessories for your head—like scarves, hats, or turbans—that do not fit too tight or feel rough and scratchy against the scalp.

## Chemobrain

Chemobrain, also referred to as cognitive dysfunction, is a symptom reported by many cancer patients. Chemobrain is a condition that makes it difficult to efficiently process information. It may be caused by the cancer itself, the chemotherapy treatment, or a secondary medical condition like anemia. Cancer patients dealing with chemobrain may find it tough to concentrate on a single task, misplace objects, have issues with short-term memory, struggle with remembering details like dates or correct words, and simply feel mentally slower than normal.

The symptoms of chemobrain will usually fade after chemotherapy treatment ends, but this varies per patient. Some individuals may notice that it takes a year or more after treatment before chemobrain symptoms are completely gone; others may never regain their full cognitive function.

Tips for dealing with chemobrain include:

- Use memory aids such as notebooks, lists, planners, or a small hand-held recorder to help keep track of events and other important information.
- Include light to moderate exercise in your day. Even 10 minutes of physical activity may help improve mental function.
- Manage other conditions like fatigue/sleep issues and depression/anxiety that can exacerbate chemobrain symptoms.
- Minimize surrounding distractions to improve concentration when you are working or trying to recall information.
- Talk to your physician about any changes that you notice in your thinking for possible referral to a neuropsychologist for further assistance.

You can contact these national organizations to learn more about cancer, ask specific questions, or receive additional data related to cancer and cancer treatments:

**American Cancer Society**
Website: www.cancer.org
Toll-free phone number: (800) 227-2345

**American Institute for Cancer Research**
Website: www.aicr.org
Toll-free phone number: (800) 843-8114

**American Society of Clinical Oncology (ASCO)**
Website: www.cancer.net
Toll-free phone number: 888-651-3038

**National Cancer Institute at the National Institutes of Health**
Website: www.cancer.gov
Toll-free phone number: 1-800-4-CANCER (1-800-422-6237)

**National Foundation for Cancer Research**
Website: www.nfcr.org
Toll-free phone number: 1-800-321-CURE (1-800-321-2873)

## Most Common Types of Cancer Diagnosed in the United States in 2014

The following is a list, compiled by the National Cancer Institute, collecting the common cancer types that were diagnosed with the greatest frequency in America (excluding non-melanoma skin cancers) in 2014:

Bladder cancer
Breast cancer
Colon and rectal cancer
Endometrial cancer
Kidney cancer
Leukemia

Lung cancer
Melanoma
Non-Hodgkin lymphoma
Pancreatic cancer
Prostate cancer
Thyroid cancer

Statistics from the American Cancer Society were used to determine the common cancer types for the list. To qualify, the estimated annual incidence for 2014 had to be 40,000 cases or more.

# CHAPTER TWO

# Improve Your Wellness Through Exercise

Individuals who deal with daily fatigue, nausea, and other painful symptoms associated with cancer may not feel very eager when it comes to exercising and engaging in physical activity. It seems to go against logic—to exercise more when you are already in pain and feeling exhausted. Yet the reality is that too much inactivity can lead to muscle weakness, reduced range of motion, and loss of body function. Physicians and researchers now support the view that certain exercises—customized to fit individual needs—can *benefit* people with cancer, instead of exacerbating their symptoms.

## How Does Exercise Benefit People Living with Cancer?

Regular exercise boosts the body's endorphins (pain-fighting molecules) and serotonin (the brain chemical that influences moods). An increase in one or both helps to naturally relieve the stress, anxiety, and depression that are often symptomatic in individuals with a chronic illness like cancer. Engaging in exercise also helps to improve moods, attitude, and quality of life for these individuals.

Other ways exercise can benefit people with cancer:
- Reduces fatigue
- Improves balance (which lowers risks of injuries and/or broken bones due to falls)
- Controls weight and burns calories
- Boosts energy levels
- Lessens nausea
- Increases aerobic ability
- Helps with quality of sleep
- Improves cardiovascular health and lowers risks of developing heart disease
- Relieves pain
- Improves blood flow to your legs (which lowers the risk of forming blood clots)
- Boosts muscle endurance and strength (and keeps them from wasting away due to inactivity)
- Improves self-esteem and positive attitudes

## What New Research Says About Exercise and Cancer Survivors

Scientific research suggests that physical activity after being diagnosed with cancer may be beneficial in improving the quality of life of the patient, while minimizing some of the side effects of the disease and treatments. Regular exercise is also linked to a reduced risk of cancer recurrence.

One study, published in the *International Journal of Sports Medicine* in 2011, examined the influence of physical activity and oxidative stress on cancer patients. Oxidative stress—a disturbance in the balance between the production of reactive oxygen species (free radicals) and antioxidant defenses—is believed to be an important factor in the onset, progression, and recurrence of cancer. In the study, researchers measured oxidative stress rates of women with breast cancer and men with prostate cancer before and after hiking. The study concluded that long-distance hiking trips may improve anti-oxidative capacity, which helps combat disease, in the blood of cancer patients.

Another study showed that breast cancer survivors who exercised regularly (the equivalent of walking 3–5 hours per week at an average pace) after a diagnosis of breast cancer had improved survival rates compared with less active women.

In the latest report from the Continuous Update Project (CUP), an analysis of 85 separate studies of over 160,000 women revealed growing evidence of links between physical activity, a healthy BMI, diet, and breast cancer mortality and subsequent primary breast cancer incidences.

CUP Panel lead and researcher at the Fred Hutchinson Cancer Research Center in Seattle, Anne McTiernan, MD, PhD, explained "[T]he research suggests that women who have a healthy weight and are physically active, both before and after they are diagnosed, have a better chance of surviving a diagnosis of breast cancer and of not getting a second primary breast cancer."

Two additional studies show a positive association of exercise after colon cancer diagnosis and survival. Participants with higher levels of physical activity post-diagnosis were proven less likely to have a cancer recurrence and had increased survival rates.

## What Kinds of Exercises Are Best for Helping with Cancer Symptoms?

The exercises found in Chapter 4 are aimed at increasing flexibility, balance, strength, stability, and mobility for people living with cancer. Combined with the carefully planned exercise programs and progressions in Chapter 5, these exercises will help to reduce symptoms and provide individuals some control over cancer pain.

On the following page are a few recommended exercises for each of the most common symptoms of cancer and cancer treatment. (Please refer to Chapter 4 for a complete list and descriptions of the exercises.)

Please remember that practicing moderation and pacing yourself are always important whenever beginning a new exercise routine. Keep in mind that, even if you exercised regularly before treatment, you may still need to exercise less or at a lower intensity during treatment. The goal is to stay as active as possible, while *slowly* increasing your exercise time and intensity only when your body is ready for it. Pay attention to your symptoms and take breaks when you need to, but don't give up. The payoff will be more energy, less pain, and a better quality of life.

**To Improve Mobility:**
Getting up from a Chair (page 27)
Getting up from the Ground (page 29)
Thoracic Flex on Roller (page 37)

**To Improve Balance:**
Standing on Toes (page 66)
Physio-Ball Foot Lifts (page 67)
Band Pulls with One Knee Up (page 73)

**To Improve Stability:**
Chair Sit (page 31)
Deadbug (page 34)
Chopping Movements (page 62)
Lifting Movements (page 63)

**To Improve Flexibility:**
Lateral Neck Stretch (page 49)
Chair Stretch (page 51)
Straight Leg Stretch (page 52)

**To Improve Strength:**
Kegel (page 65)
Open Hip Squats (page 54)
Alphabet Series: T's (page 39)
Alphabet Series: W's (page 40)
Alphabet Series: Y's (page 41)

# CHAPTER THREE

---

# Rules of the Road:
# Exercise Precautions

In the next chapter, you will find many great exercises, designed to satisfy cancer patients' need for physical activity, including exercises that improve balance, strength, and mobility. The exercises and programs found in Chapters 4 and 5 are specially designed to be safe and effective, even for those with recurring pain.

Patients following the programs in Chapter 5 should not hesitate to cater the program to their own specific needs and abilities by substituting the exercises that they really enjoy. You'll be more likely to complete your exercise programs with increased regularity and consistency when they are made up of exercises that you enjoy. Remember that regularity *and* consistency both are the two key factors for achieving a healthier body.

In performing these exercises, you will be participating in something called *motor learning*. It is important to keep in mind that there will be a learning curve for new physical and mental exercises, which may cause some frustration as you become accustomed to the new movements and activities.

The first few weeks of the program are called the *cognitive (or verbal) stage,* during which you will be mentally figuring out what to do. This should last three to four weeks.

During the second learning stage, named the *associative stage,* you should be able to perform the action, but possibly with some errors. This should last two to three weeks.

Finally, the *automatic stage* is when you are able to perform the exercises without error (or with "great form") and can repeat sets and reps week after week.

## Exercise Essentials Checklist

### Exercise Preparation

- **Exercise Location:** Is your environment safe, clean, and free of debris?
- **Proper Footwear:** Are you wearing proper athletic footwear?
- **Comfortable Athletic Wear:** Do you have clothes that allow freedom of movement?
- **Hydration:** Be sure to drink six glasses of fluid over the course of your day.

### Exercise Equipment

- **Rolled-up towel:** Can be used for resistance training, balancing on the floor, etc.
- **Mirror:** Provides visual feedback on cueing and technique
- **Dumbbells:** 5–10 pound range is generally appropriate
- **Therabands:** Light-colored bands offer less resistance and dark-colored bands offer more resistance
- **Physio-ball:** Inflate the ball to the point where you can press your thumb on the surface without it sinking in
- **Tennis ball or racquet ball:** For hand and foot therapy

## Playing it Safe: Important Safety Precautions

The following are some helpful tips and safety practices to observe when exercising. Read them over carefully, and make them a part of your learning process. Note that the most important safety precaution is making sure to see your healthcare provider regularly for check-ups.

**Body Positioning:** Brace your core, achieve proper alignment, feel the placement of your feet, and always move first from your core before moving your limbs.

**Keep a Health Journal:** Record how you're feeling on any given day, along with the activities you did during that time. You should also record what kinds of exercises you did on each day, and how you felt both during and after your exercise session. Keeping track of this information will help you better understand your own health, which is a crucial step on the road to recovery.

**Rate of Perceived Exertion (RPE):** You can use the chart below to gauge how hard you are working during your session. The corresponding numerical values may also be helpful for you to record in your Health Journal, should you choose to keep one.

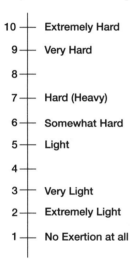

10 — Extremely Hard

9 — Very Hard

8 —

7 — Hard (Heavy)

6 — Somewhat Hard

5 — Light

4 —

3 — Very Light

2 — Extremely Light

1 — No Exertion at all

**Talk Test:** This is another useful way of determining how hard you are working. As you are exercising, gauge how easily you are able to converse and use the guidelines below to figure out the intensity of your exertion.

If you can carry on a normal conversation while exercising, you are likely working *aerobically,* which means your body is using oxygen as its primary energy source. If you can work aerobically for up to 30–45 minutes, your body will also be using fat as an energy source, which is an excellent foundation for building your exercise program.

*Anaerobic work,* characterized below as medium intensity, should be introduced eight weeks into your exercise program. Examples include hill walking, bike sprints, etc. When performing anaerobic exercise, you may notice your leg muscles starting to feel a bit tight, your chest will expand, you will begin to sweat, and your heart rate will reach about 40–50 beats above your resting heart rate (see the next page for more details on determining your heart rate).

**Low Intensity**: Complete sentences, breathing rate normal
**Medium Intensity:** Broken sentences, breathing rate slightly labored
**High Intensity:** Cannot converse, breathing rate labored

### *Determining Your Heart Rate*

To determine your heart rate, place the tips of your index, second and third fingers on your wrist, below the base of your thumb. You can also place the tips of your index and second fingers on your neck, along either side of your windpipe. During exercise, it is recommended that you find your pulse on your wrist, rather than on your neck.

When pressing lightly with your fingers, you should be able to feel your pulse. If you don't feel your pulse, move your fingers around slightly until you find your pulse. Count the number of beats you feel in 10 seconds. Using that number, calculate your heart rate with the formula below:

**(Beats in ten seconds) x 6 = (Heart Rate)**

Adults over 18 years of age typically have a resting heart rate of 60–100 beats per minute. To better understand your own heart rate, you should check your pulse both before and immediately after exercising. This will give you a better idea of what your body normally does at rest, and what level your heart should be working at during an exercise session.

## Calculating Target Heart Rate

Your target heart rate is the level of exertion you should aim for when exercising in order to gain the most benefits from your workout. Your target heart rate is also a useful range for how your body is responding to your workout.

Target heart rate is 60-80% of your maximum heart rate, depending on what level of exertion you wish to work at.

**Different Training Zones**

Below is a list of the different levels of exertion and the corresponding percentage you would use to target heart rate:

*Recovery Zone - 60% to 70%*
Active recovery training should fall into this zone (ideally at the lower end). It's also useful for very early pre-season and closed season cross training when the body needs to recover and replenish.

*Aerobic Zone - 70% to 80%*
Exercising in this zone will help to develop your aerobic system and, in particular, your ability to transport and utilize oxygen. Continuous or rhythmic endurance training, like running and hiking, should fall under this heart rate zone.

*Anaerobic Zone – 80% to 90%*
Training in this zone will help to improve your body's ability to deal with lactic acid. It may also help to increase your lactate threshold.

To determine your target heart rate, you can use the formulas below to calculate your maximum heart rate, and to then find your target heart rate.

**220 – age = maximum heart rate**
**Maximum heart rate x training % = target heart rate**

For example, if a 50 year old woman wishes to train at 70% of her maximum heart rate, she would use the below calculations:

**220 – 50 = 170**
**170 x 70% = 119**

She would thus aim to reach a heart rate of 119 during her exercise in order to work at her target heart rate.

You can also use the Karvonen Formula, which is based on both maximum heart rate and resting heart. Visit www.sport-fitnessadvisor.com/heart-rate-reserve.html for more information.

## Don't Discount Your Blood Counts

Cancer and the types of chemotherapy and other drugs used to fight cancer can often affect the blood cell counts in your body. Your blood counts should be monitored regularly at your treatment sessions and doctor's visits. It is important to always be aware if your blood counts are at safe levels, as well as ensuring that they remain at safe levels when you are active in an exercise program.

- **White blood cells (WBCs)** protect your body from infection by attacking invading bacteria, viruses, and other foreign materials in the body. If you have a low white blood cell count or take medications that reduce your ability to fight infections, it is advisable to avoid exercising in public gyms until your counts return to a safe level.

- **Red blood cells (RBCs)** carry oxygen throughout your body. You may not be able to safely participate in an exercise program if you have a low red blood cell count (known as anemia), so be sure to have your red blood cell count checked regularly and discuss physical activity options with your physician.

- **Platelets** help to stop bleeding by forming blood clots. Patients with low platelet levels have a greater risk of serious bruising or bleeding, so use extreme caution when engaging in physical activity or refrain until your counts are normal again.

## Important Assessments

### *Medical Tests*

Medical tests, including blood panels, neurological/reflexive tests, updated family history, and stress tests are tests that your medical provider can provide based upon their clinical assessment of your health and risk profile. Maintain an open dialogue with your medical practitioner, particularly if you or your family has a history of heart problems.

### *Fitness Tests (Functional and Physical Assessments)*

**Functional Assessment:** The Functional Assessment will provide you with a direct measurement of how you can improve in your daily activities. This includes walking stairs, getting in and out of chairs, etc. Refer to Chapter 5, page 91 for the Functional Assessment.

**Physical Assessment:** The Physical Assessment will provide you with a direct measurement of the improvements you can make in gaining strength as a result of following the exercises in this book. Refer to Chapter 5, page 91 for the Physical Assessment.

**Waist Size:** To determine your waist-to-height ratio, simply divide your waist size by your height (in inches). A waist-to-height ratio under 50 percent is generally considered healthy.

**Stamina:** The average person should be able to walk up a flight of stairs or walk once around an outdoor track without becoming out of breath.

**12-Minute Walking Test:** Find a measured distance, such as a track, and see how much distance you can cover in 12 minutes. (You can complete this on a treadmill, too.) Make sure you challenge yourself, while still being able to carry on intermittent conversation with a partner (see the Talk Test on page 19).

Refer to the Rate of Perceived Exertion (RPE) scale on page 19. You should aim to work at around 5–6 during the first two or three repetitions of this test. Thereafter, challenge yourself to reach a 7–8 on the RPE scale. This test is also known as the Cooper Test.

**Quarter-Mile Timed Test:** Find a measured 400-meter or quarter-mile track. See how long it takes you to cover the specified distance. Aim to work at a 6–7 on the Rate of Perceived Exertion (RPE) scale.

**Strength:** As you perform Strength Circuits (see pages 96-98), make note of any improvements you have made. For instance, are you able to perform more reps? Have you continued on from beginner to intermediate exercises?

**Flexibility:** Because levels of flexibility can differ greatly from one individual to the next, it is impossible to provide an average measurement of flexibility. Instead, you should aim to determine what improvements you are seeing in your Physical Assessment (see page 91) from week to week. This will help you gauge whether you are improving your flexibility (based on your body's abilities).

**Re-Assessment:** Perform the Functional Assessment and Physical Assessment again and compare your new results with your original results to determine how much you have improved in your overall strength and function.

# CHAPTER FOUR

# The Exercises

# Stair Walking

## Feel it Here Back

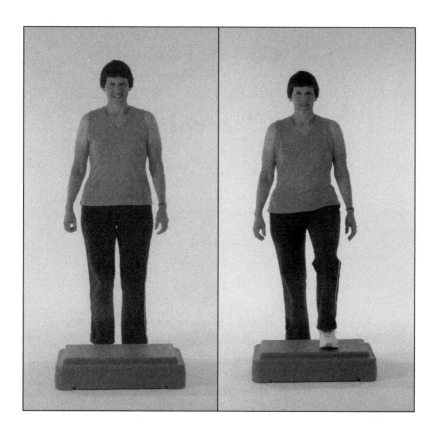

**SET-UP**

Position yourself in front of a set of stairs, with your feet hip-width apart. Place one foot on the first step. Press the foot into the step to engage your hip and lower back muscles. Use the railing until you get stronger. Feel the full foot pressing into the step without letting the hips slide to the side.

# Getting Up From a Chair
## Feel it Here Core

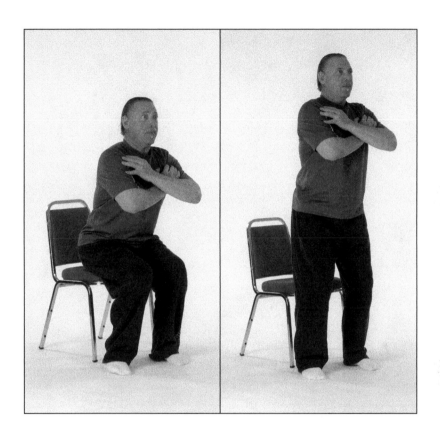

**SET-UP**

Position yourself on the edge of a chair. Hips should be parallel, or slightly above, knee level. Brace your core and press your feet into the ground.

# Standing with Eyes Closed

## Feel it Here Full Body

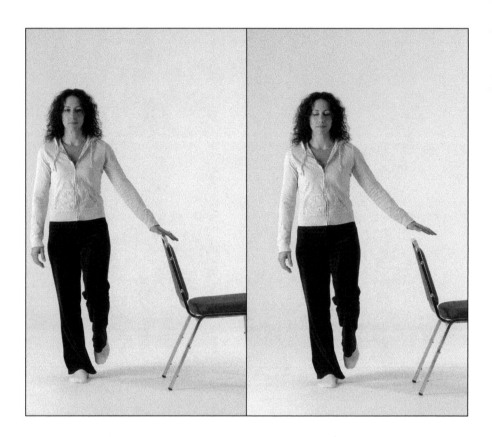

**SET-UP**

Stand with your feet hip-width apart. You should stand near a wall or partner for safety. For the two-legged test, rest you hands at your side and close your eyes. With both feet on the ground, feel a natural sway similar to a tree in the wind. For the one-legged test, close your eyes once your foot is off the ground. With one foot on the ground, the sway will increase dramatically with your body wanting to make very quick readjustments to stabilize.

# Getting up from the Ground

## Feel it Here Core, Shoulders, Legs

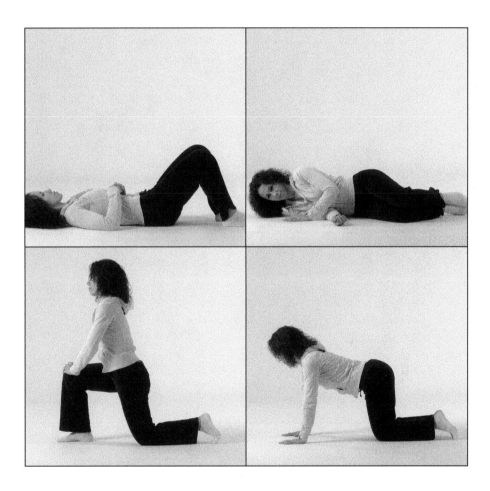

## SET-UP

Position yourself on your back or stomach, with your hands above your shoulders. Brace your stomach. Move your torso first and naturally. Allow your body segments to follow into an all fours position. You should be near a wall or couch in case you need assistance getting up.

*Images should be read clockwise.*

# Ribs Heavy

## Feel it Here Lower Ribs, Abs

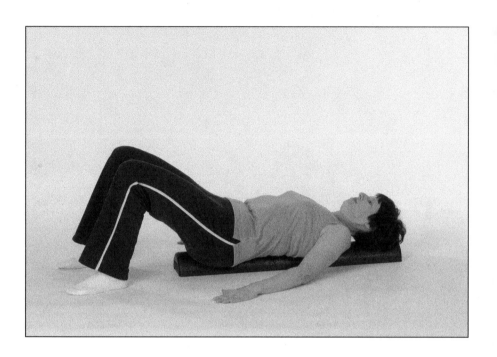

**SET-UP**

Use a foam roller or towel rolled up lengthwise. Make sure your head, middle back, and hips are in contact with the roller or towel. Feel your lower ribs make contact with the roller, yet make sure you have space in your lower back. This movement replaces pushing your lower back into the ground or flattening out your lower back during core movements, and will be applied to all exercises. When lying on your back, the body should contact the floor at your head, shoulders, hips, upper legs and calves. Your neck, lower back, and space behind your knees should be off the floor.

# Chair Sit

## Feel it Here Legs

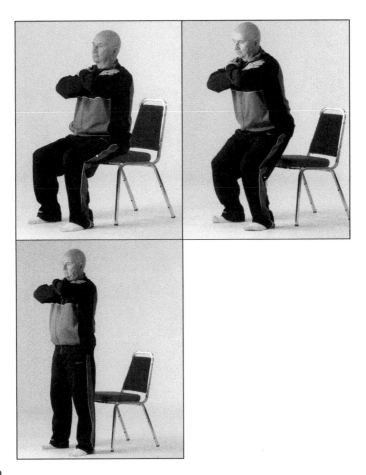

## SET-UP

Using the chair as a teaching tool, lift the hips off the seat using legs and hips. Hold this position, relax into the chair, repeat. Work on increasing the time held for each rep. A wall can be used if the isometric squat is too much. Position your body against a wall. Walk your hips down the wall by walking your feet out in front of your body. Keep your hips, knees, and toes in line. Maintaining head, shoulder, and tailbone contact with the wall, hold the squatting position as if sitting in a chair. You should not feel pain in your knees. If you do, walk the feet out farther. Breathe into your lower body.

# Forward Plank

**Feel it Here**  Stomach, Legs, Shoulders

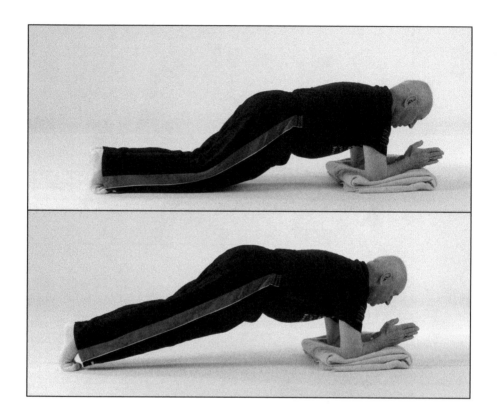

**SET-UP**

Position your body in the same position as a push-up, but with your hands positioned together in front of your face. To help cue the pulling of the navel to the spine, place a rolled-up towel on your lower back as a bio-feedback tool. Make sure you are breathing through the entire movement. Pull your navel to the lower spine but do not flatten out your lower back. Instead, cue the lower ribs to become "heavy."

# Lateral Plank

## Feel it Here Stomach, Legs, Shoulders

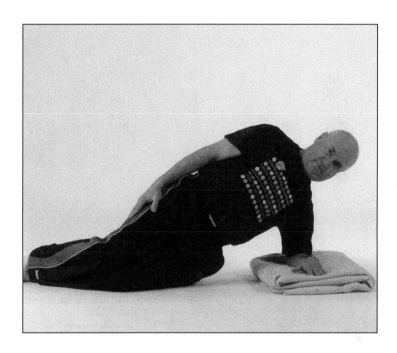

**SET-UP**
Position you body on one side, on your elbow and hip. Contract the side of your stomach and elevate your hip into alignment with the shoulders and knees.

# Deadbug

## Feel it Here Core, Arms, Legs

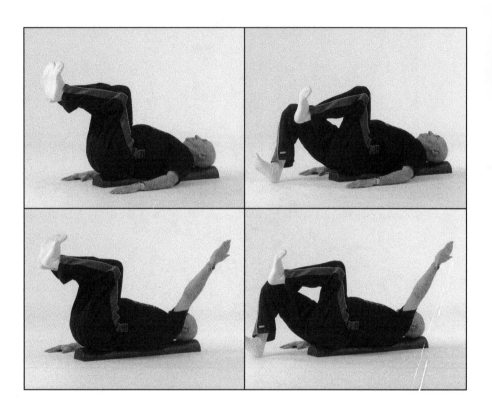

**SET-UP**

Beginning on your back, practice bracing your stomach with a 'marble squeeze' in the navel and combine that with a kegel (see page 65). Position a towel under your lumbar spine as a feedback tool to maintaining a neutral, not a flat, back spine. Draw one leg out with your spine neutral. Try both legs. Focus on your core contact maintaining neutral spine during arm and leg movements.

*Images should be read clockwise.*

# Hip Hinging

**Feel it Here** Lower Spine, Hamstrings

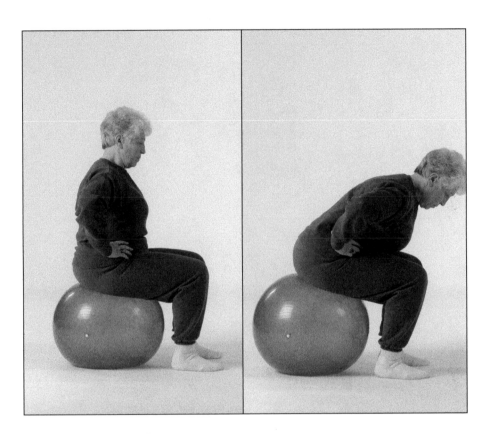

## SET-UP

Start the movement from your hips, letting the other parts follow. Feel your upper body positioned over the upper thighs as you "hinge" forward. Brace your stomach, then begin the upward movement, returning to an upright position.

# Spinal Whip

**Feel it Here** Middle Back

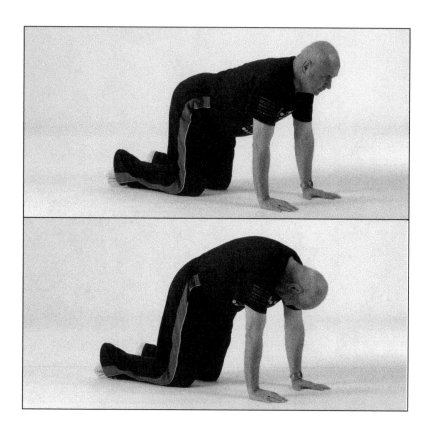

### SET-UP

Begin on all fours or standing with your hands on your knees. Rotate from the shoulder blades as they move to the outside of the upper body. Emphasize moving from the middle back through the sternum.

**Note:** Pay special attention to noticing the difference between your lower, middle, and upper back.

# Thoracic Flex on Roller

**Feel it Here** Middle Spine, Abdominals

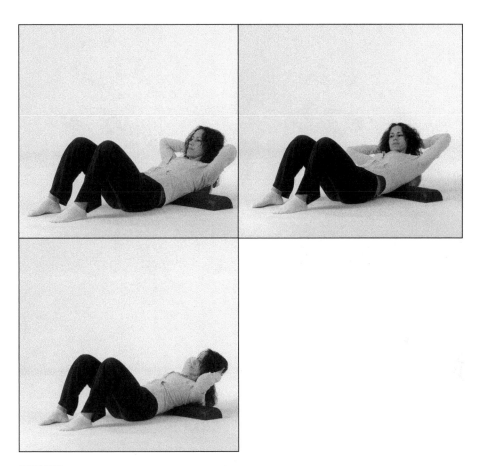

**SET-UP**

You can use a full roller, half roller, or thick, rolled-up towel. Position the roller immediately below your shoulder blades. Your elbows should be pointed to the sides. Feel the foam roller pressing against your middle spine. Keep your ribs heavy into the ground so the core muscles are active and working through the entire motion. Your front abs will be working the entire time but the latter muscles, namely the obliques, are the actual movers.

**Note:** This should be attempted using a half roller first and then using a full roller.

# Ribcage Opener

## Feel it Here Groin, Back, Shoulders

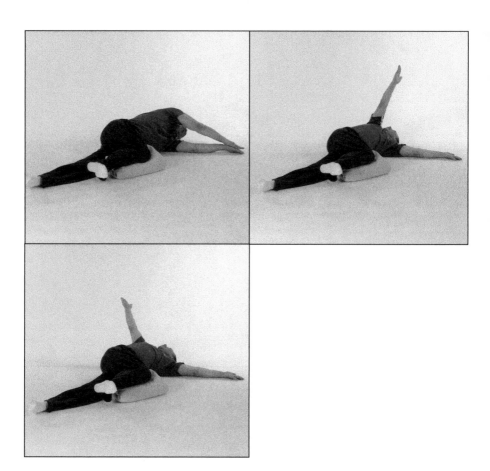

**SET-UP**

Lay on the ground and position a rolled-up towel or foam roller under your knee. Start with your hands together. Press your knees into the object, then initiate rotation with your hand. Follow the rotation down the arm until you feel it through your ribcage.

# Alphabet Series: T's

**Feel it Here** Middle Back, Behind Shoulders

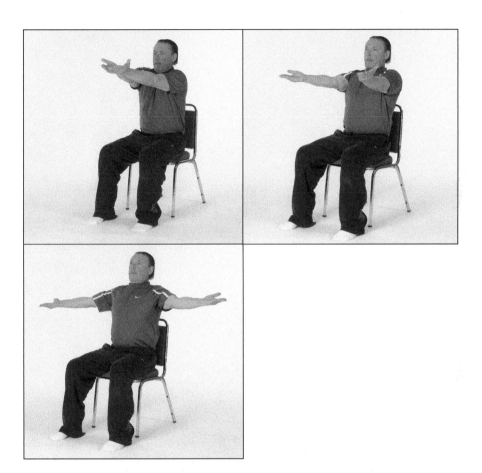

**SET-UP**

Sit upright on a sturdy surface. Squeeze your shoulder blades back and down. Draw both arms out from the mid-line of the body with palms up.

# Alphabet Series: W's

## Feel it Here Middle Back

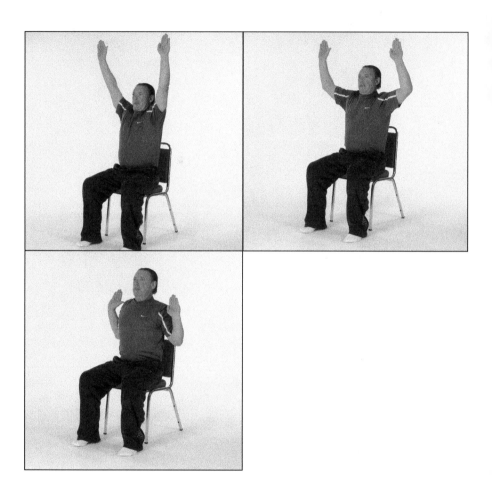

**SET-UP**
Sit upright on a sturdy surface. Squeeze your shoulder blades back and down. Draw both elbows down and back into the middle spine. Hold, then release.

# Alphabet Series: Y's

**Feel it Here**  Middle and Lower Back

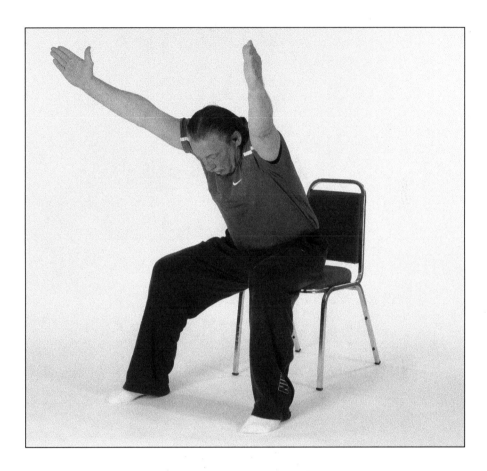

**SET-UP**

Sit upright on a sturdy surface.  Squeeze your shoulder blades back and down.  Draw both arms up and straight out in front of your body at a 45 degree angle.

# Cranial Release

## Feel it Here Neck

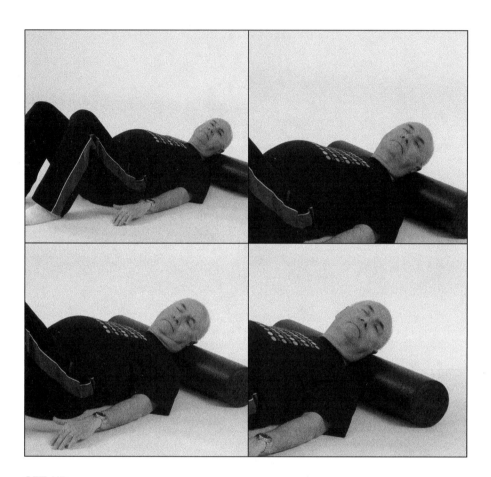

**SET-UP**

Lay on your back. Position the back of your head, right where it meets the base of your neck, on the roller. You should be in a comfortable position; draw your feet into your hips if needed. Your hands should be relaxed near the sides of your hips. If you need to stabilize the roller, place your hands on the sides of the roller. Rotate your head to the right and left. When rotating your head to the right and left, feel the small space that sits on either side of your head. Keep pressure in the roller by slightly extending your neck, emphasizing proper alignment. *Check out www.meltmethod.com*

*Images should be read clockwise.*

42

# Glutes

**Feel it Here** Outer Hip, Lower Back, Hamstrings

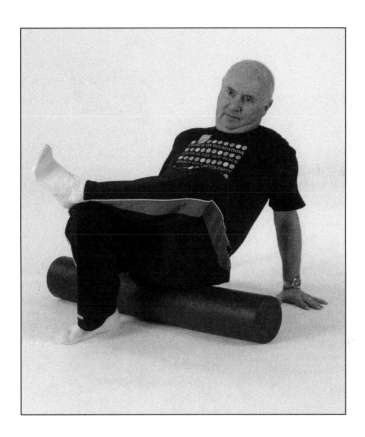

**SET-UP**
Position your outer hip on the roller. Apply pressure into the roller with the hip, and slowly rotate the hip from the knee.

# Sacral Release

## Feel it Here Pelvis

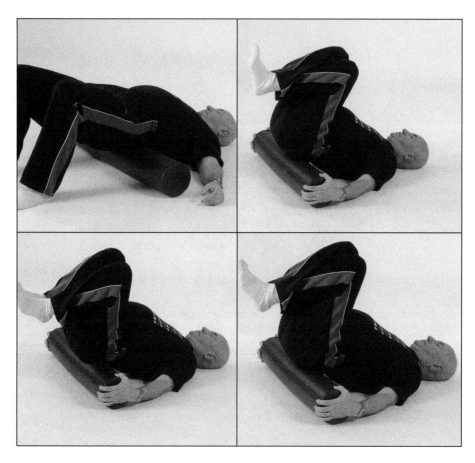

**SET-UP**

Position your body in a comfortable bridging position on your spine. Elevate your hips and slide the roller on your sacrum. Keeping your ribs heavy, engaging your core, pull one knee at a time up to a position over your hips. Addressing one side of your pelvis at a time, let your knees drift over until you feel a "barrier" or place of irritability. Once found, gently make circles with your knees both ways, then switch to the other side.

*Check out www.meltmethod.com*

*Images should be read clockwise.*

# Lateral Side Bend on Physio-Ball

**Feel it Here** Ribcage, Shoulders, Lower Back

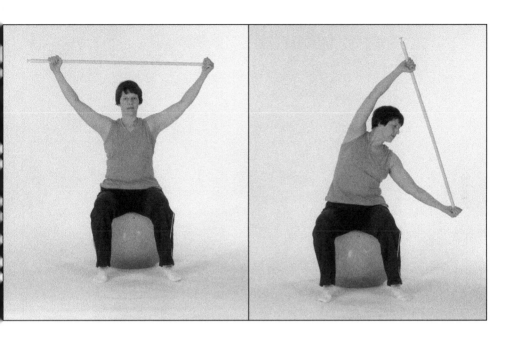

**SET-UP**

Sitting atop the physio-ball, maintain a stance wider than hip-width. Push the broomstick above the head with straight arms. Initiating the motion from the hands, slowly flex the back to one side. The stick will be cupped into the bottom hand. If your opposite hip comes up, you have gone too far.

# Adductors with Band

## Feel it Here Inner Groin, Hip

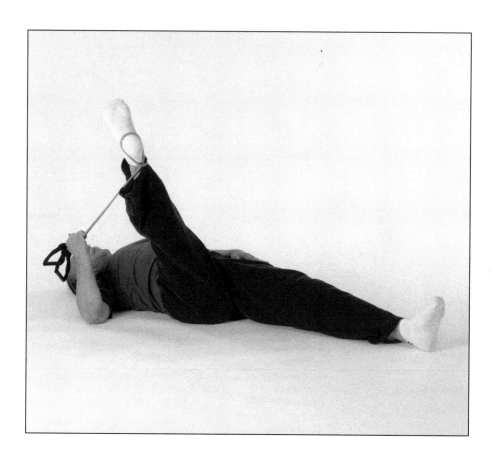

**SET-UP**

Wrap the towel or stretch cord around the ankle of the leg you want to stretch. Keeping the non-stretching leg down on the floor, press your ankle in toward your body against resistance, and release. Hold the pressure for five seconds. Release and breathe out slowly. Repeat the movement from the newly obtained position.

# Quads/Hip Flexors

**Feel it Here** Front of Leg

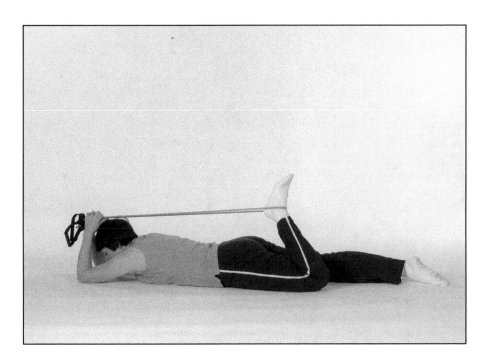

### SET-UP

This exercise can be done lying on your stomach or on your side. Lying on your stomach decreases the likelihood that you will arch your lower back during the stretch. Hold the pressure for 5 seconds, then release and breathe out slowly. Repeat the movement from the newly obtained position. If you are feeling the stretch in your lower back, place a pillow or rolled-up towel under the front of your hips for support. If you are feeling the stretch in the front of your knee, place the towel under the front of your knee and continue with the stretch.

# Kneeling with Hand Across Knee

**Feel it Here** Middle & Lower Back, Hips, Chest, Shoulders

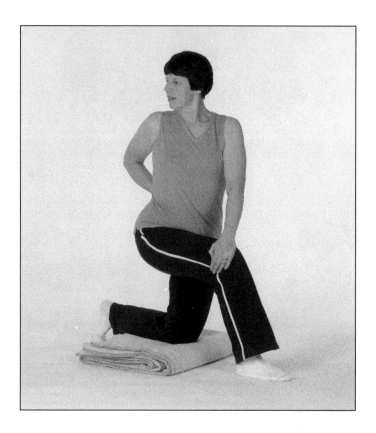

**SET-UP**

Find an elevated surface such as a step or bench. Place your foot onto the surface keeping your ankle, knee, and hip in-line. Stand as upright as possible, emphasizing rotation through your middle (not the lower) back. Place your hand across your knee to assist in rotation.

# Lateral Neck Stretch

## Feel it Here Neck, Shoulder

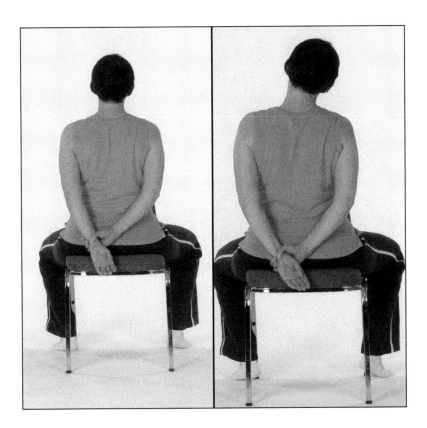

**SET-UP**

Sit with the arm of the shoulder to be stretched placed behind you. Gently drop your ear to your other shoulder. Then, grab the wrist of the shoulder/ neck area being stretched and hold. Relax the opposite shoulder by breathing deeply into the side being stretched. Allow your head to return to neutral before releasing the wrist.

# Knee to Forehead

## Feel it Here Hips

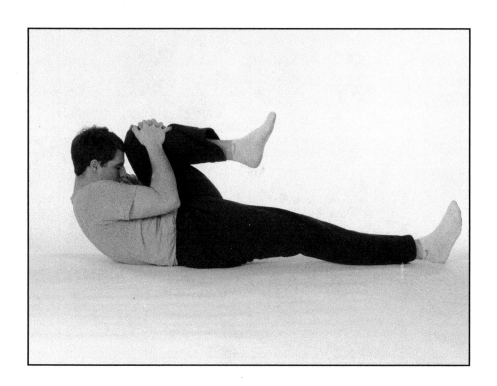

**SET-UP**
Tighten up the stomach. Draw the knee towards the chest, grabbing the knee with two hands.

# Chair Stretch

## Feel it Here Groin, Hips

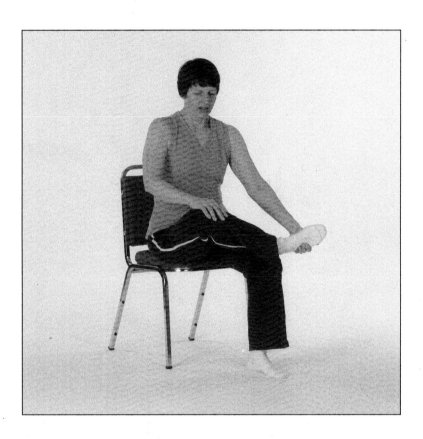

**SET-UP**

Sit upright with your hips at the same height as the knees. Breathe out and release the pressure. Pause, then assist the knees out farther. For additional support, sit against a chair back. Make sure the non-stretching hip stays firmly planted in the seat.

# Straight Leg Stretch

**Feel it Here** Back of Leg

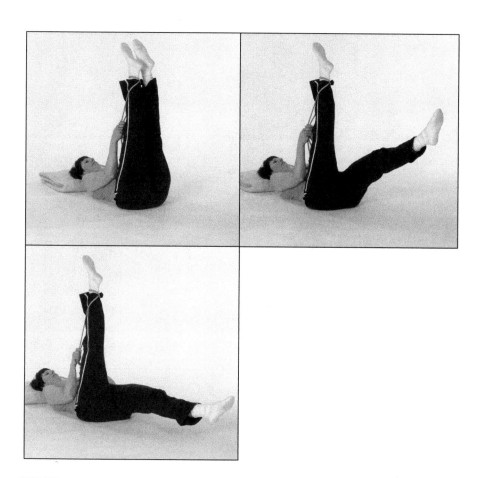

**SET-UP**

This stretch can be done using a door frame or stretch cord (as shown). Both variations are great stretches for the back of the leg.

# Ankle Pumps

## Feel it Here Front of Shins, Calves

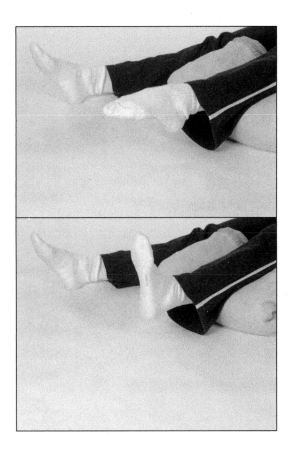

**SET-UP**

Gently point and flex the foot, reaching out through the front of the big toe.
Pull the toes back by pushing through the heel.

53

# Open Hip Squats

**Feel it Here** Groin, Hips, Legs, Lower Back

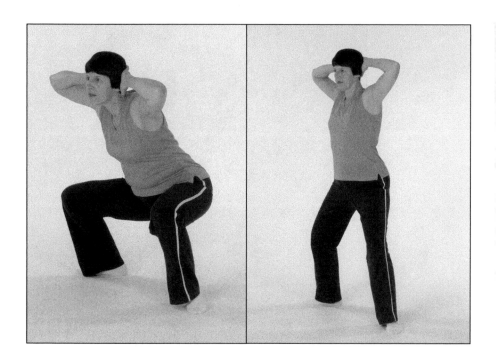

**SET-UP**

Start in a standard squatting position with your toes positioned at 11 and 1 o'clock. Keeping your back straight, initiate the opening of the hips from the legs. Drop the hips down and back into the squat.

# Hip Lifters

## **Feel it Here** Hips, Back

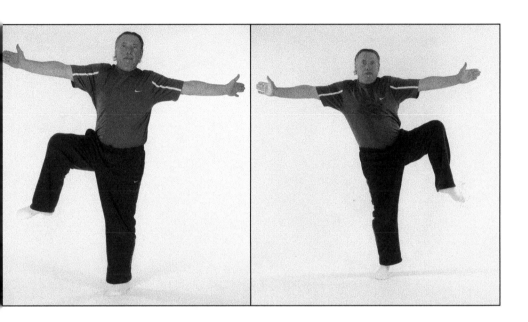

**SET-UP**

With hands out to the side, draw the hip out and knee up behind the arm.
Feel the hips and back working throughout this exercise.

55

# Physio-Ball Roll

**Feel it Here** Stomach, Ribs, Chest, Shoulders

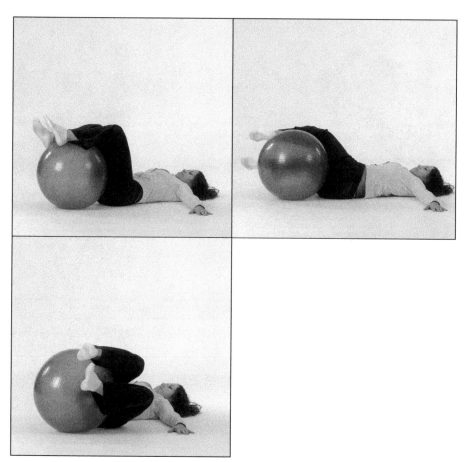

**SET-UP**

Cup your legs over a physio-ball at an angle slightly greater than 90 degrees, or a square angle at the knees and hips. Position your arms out to the side with palms down to aid in stability during lower body movement. On the way toward the floor, breathe in and gently press the back of your legs into the ball thereby slowing the legs down. On the way back to your starting position, breathe out and press your hand into the floor to activate the stomach and shoulders. This stabilizes your spine prior to moving the ball.

# Offering

**Feel it Here**  Middle Back, Shoulder Blades

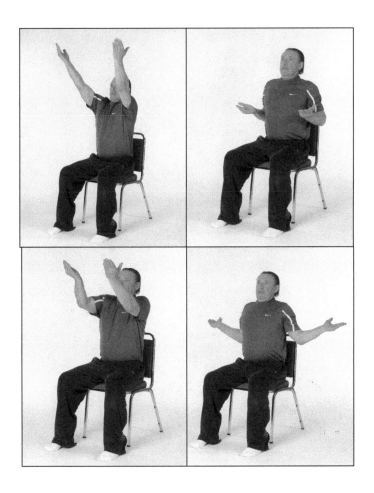

### SET-UP
Position your body in a stable sitting position with your arms extended in front of your body. Initiate movement by pulling your shoulder blades back and down. Once shoulder blades are positioned, pull your elbows back into the body and follow with an external rotation.

*Images should be read clockwise.*

# Roll and Hold

**Feel it Here** Upper and Lower Spine

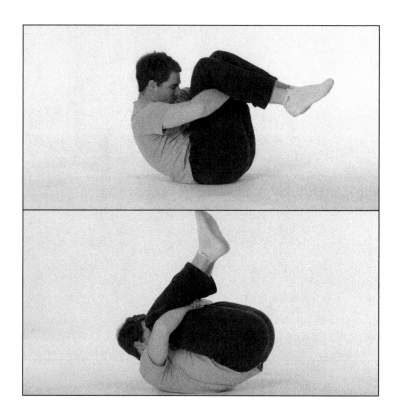

**SET-UP**
Tuck the knees into your chest and rock back and forth.

# Foam Roller Scissor Stretch

## Feel it Here  Core, Lower Back

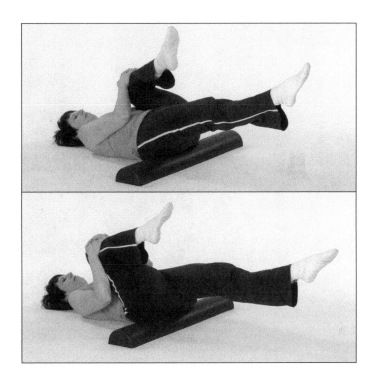

**SET-UP**

Lay on your back with your knees bent and feet close to your hips. Press your feet into the floor, then elevate your hips. Slide a foam roller (or very thick towel) beneath your tailbone/sacrum. Keeping your ribs heavy, pull one knee to your chest and hold. Extend the leg next, keeping ribs heavy and engaging the core. The sacrum is the flattish bone that positions itself directly below the lower back. Place the palm of your hand on the sacrum; it should fit nicely. The roller sits between the lower back and sacrum. *Check out www.meltmethod.com*

# Doggy Door
## Feel it Here Groin, Hips

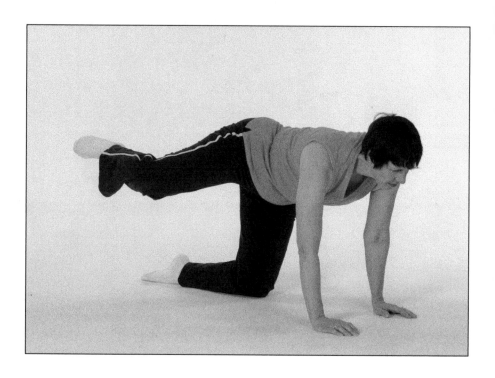

**SET-UP**

Keep you core active to stabilize your back and hips. Keeping the non-lifting hip firm into the ground, lift the opposite knee with the outside hip muscle. Be careful not to shift your weight to the non-working side.

# Pelvic Tilt

**Feel it Here** Obliques, Abdominals, Lower Back

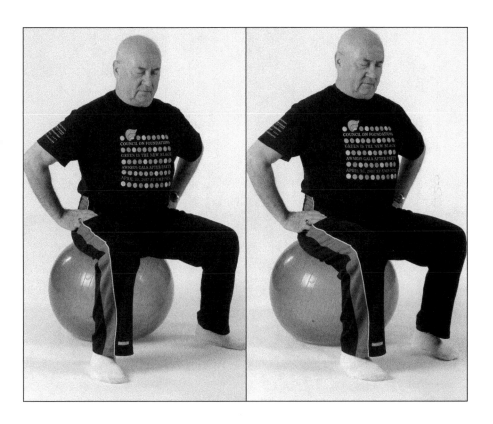

## SET-UP

Sit on a physio-ball with both knees bent and your feet flat on the floor. Tilt your pelvis in line with your hips. You may also place your hand on your belly and lower back to facilitate movement. Feel the difference between this exercise and the kegel exercise on page 65. You should notice a distinct anatomical difference between the lower back and ribs.

# Chopping Movements
## Feel it Here Core, Hips

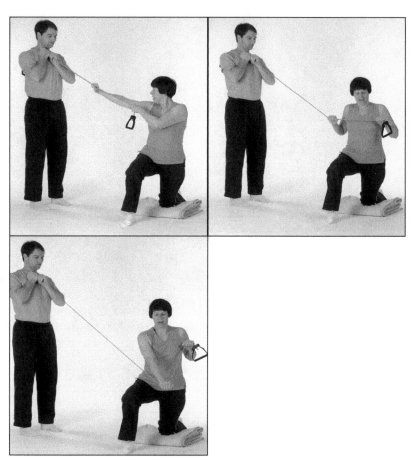

**SET-UP**

Chop across your body over a trailing, kneeling leg. Your front knee is on the ground on a towel or other comfortable item. Pull the band into your body, then push it down and out with the trail hand. Keep your spine neutral by concentrating on bracing your stomach and stabilizing the hips. Think about moving around a stable pillar in your spine.

*Exercise provided by St. John's, AAHFRP, FMS*

62

# Lifting Movements

## Feel it Here Core, Hips

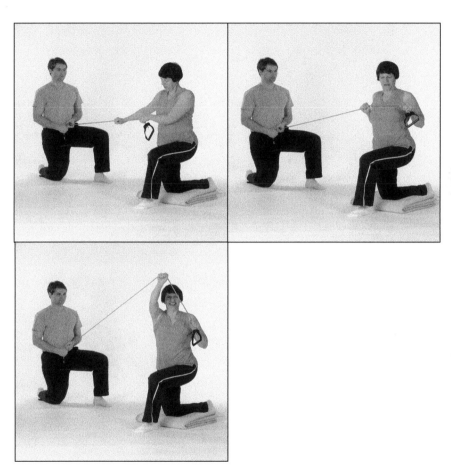

**SET-UP**

You will be lifting across your body over a trailing knee on the ground. The front knee should be aligned with your hip. Pull the band into your body, then push it up and out with the trailing hand. Keep your spine neutral by concentrating on bracing your stomach and stabilizing the hips. Think about moving around a stable pillar in your spine.

*Exercise provided by St. John's, AAHFRP, FMS*

# Prone Extension Lifts

**Feel it Here** Middle and Lower Back, Hips

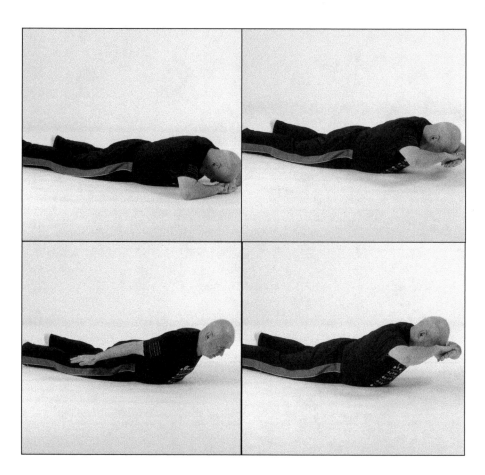

**SET-UP**

Gently press the front of your lower body into the ground. Initiate the lifting movement from your head, then shoulders, middle back, and lower back. Hold, then release slowly.

*Images should be read clockwise.*

# Kegel

**Feel it Here** Pelvic Floor, Core

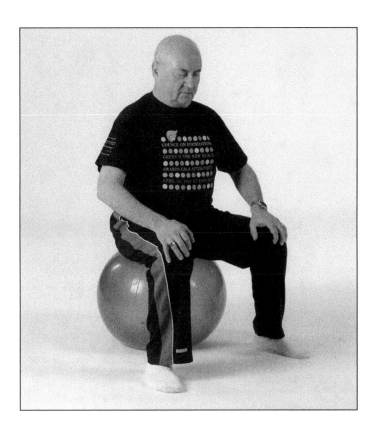

## SET-UP
While keeping the lower back quiet and relaxed, squeeze your pelvic floor muscles in and up towards the pelvis. Imagine there is a balloon attached to your pelvic floor and it is rising. Try this exercise on the floor first to take surrounding muscles out of the learning curve.

# Standing on Toes

## Feel it Here Calves

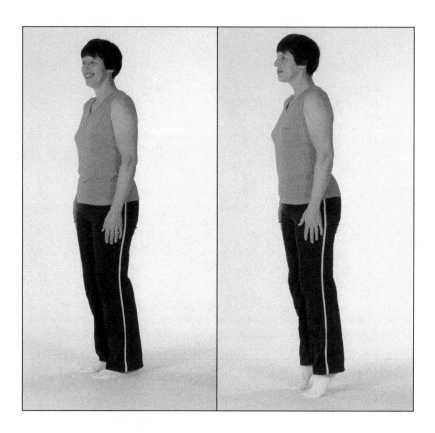

**SET-UP**

Stand with your feet parallel and pointed forward. You should be able to see the front of your feet when looking down. Lightly touch your hands against a chair or wall. Press the balls of your feet into the ground then lift your heels to the back of your hips.

# Physio-Ball Foot Lifts

## Feel it Here  Hips, Legs

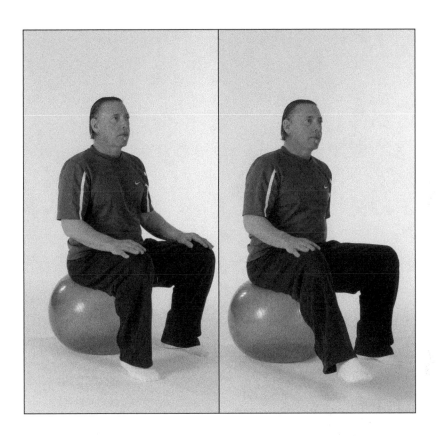

**SET-UP**

Sit on the very top of the physio-ball. You should feel as if you are sitting slightly higher than on a regular chair and a bit more open in the front of the hips. Use the hip hinging cue (see page 35) to find the back alignment necessary to maintain positioning and stability. Feel braced through the core. This will stabilize your back and hips before you lift your foot. Lift one foot off the floor, hold. Work on shifting your body weight slowly to one foot prior to lifting the opposing knee/foot. Use a mirror or partner to accomplish.

# Physio-Ball Walk-Up

## Feel it Here Legs, Hips, Core

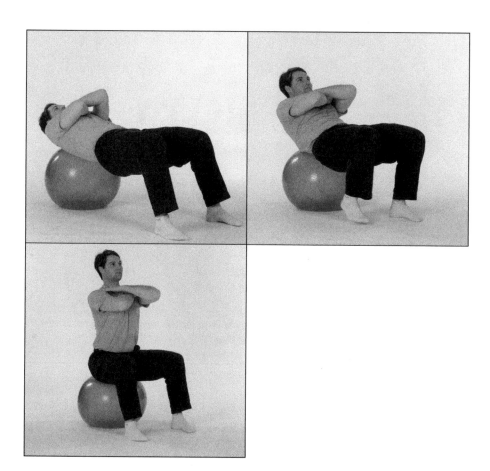

### SET-UP
Position your hips on top of the physio-ball. Brace your core. Walk up the ball using your full foot. Keeping the feet wider adds stability if you feel off balance during the up or down phases.

# Weight Shifting

## Feel it Here Hips, Legs

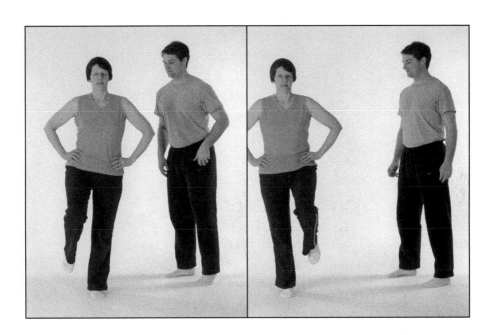

**SET-UP**

Your partner begins in normal walking position. As he or she walks forward, spot from the left to right leg, as your partner balances momentarily on each leg. Partner should feel the hips and legs working to stabilize the body during the momentary pause phase.

# Heel to Toe Rocks
## Feel it Here Full Body

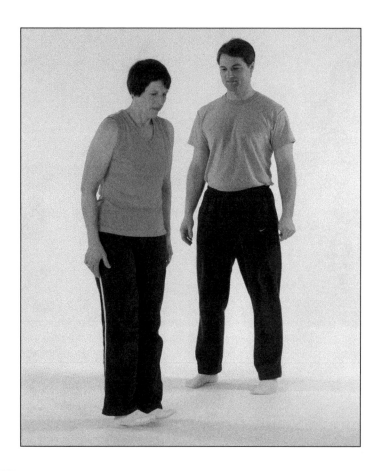

**SET-UP**

Partner rocks back and forth from the toes to heels as you provide support if needed.

# Band Presses with Two Arms

## Feel it Here  Chest, Shoulders, Arms

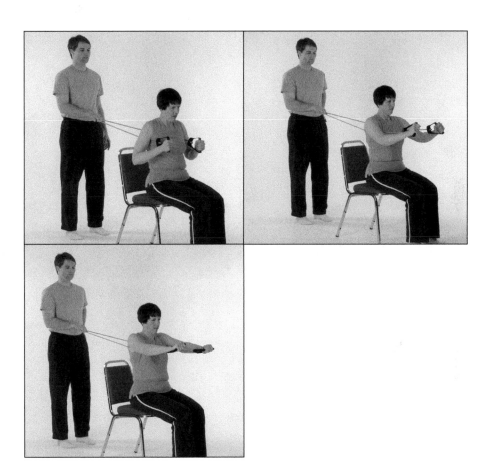

**SET-UP**

Position your body in a standing position in a normal stance or a split stance. Press your hands out in front until your elbows are fully extended. Keep the ribs heavy and core contracted during each pressing repetition. Breathe out during each extension and breathe in upon return to the starting position. This exercise can also be done while sitting (shown above) in an upright position on either a ball or a bench.

# Band Rows

**Feel it Here** Middle Back, Arms

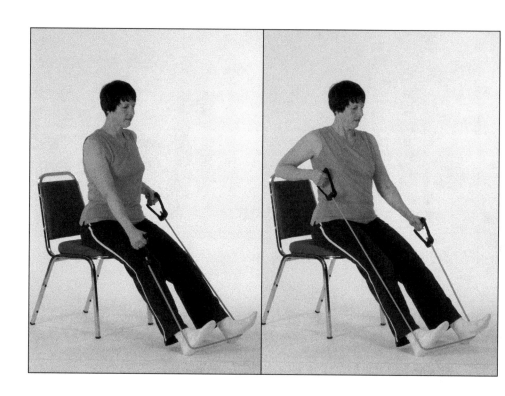

### SET-UP

Execute the movement by drawing one elbow back while "punching" the opposite arm forward. The objective is to learn rotation and build strength in the traditionally weak core and shoulder girdle. This is important for posture during walking and sitting. If you feel discomfort in your neck, concentrate on relaxing the shoulder blades back and down.

# Band Pulls with One Knee Up

**Feel it Here** Core, Arms, Chest, Legs

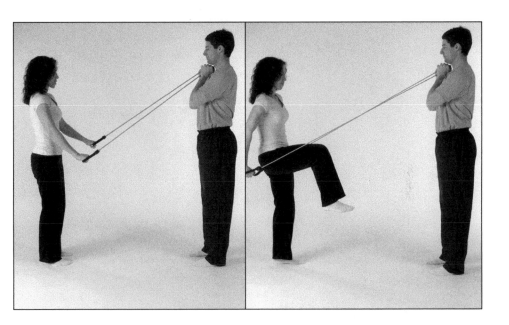

**SET-UP**

In a standing position, pull your knee upward towards your chest while pulling the arms to the sides of your body. Keep your ribs heavy and core contracted during each pressing repetition. Breathe out during each pressing rep and breathe in upon returning to the starting position.

# Row with Tricep Extension

## Feel it Here Back, Triceps

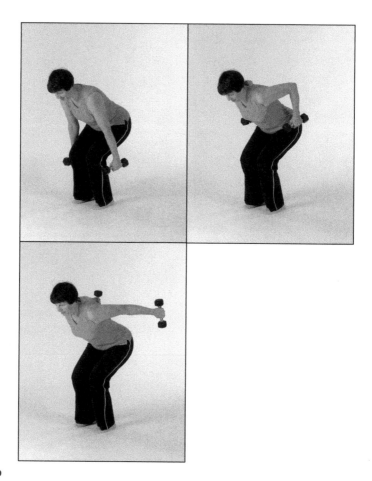

**SET-UP**

Either kneel (and use one arm) or stand and use both arms, shown above.
Perform a row, pulling your elbows behind your back and then extend your
arm fully in back of you to work the triceps.

# Single Leg Deadlift

**Feel it Here** Glutes, Hamstrings

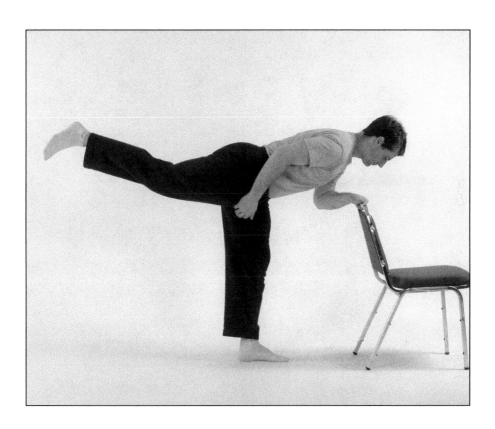

**SET-UP**
Draw one leg back straight while keeping your hips square. Perform the deadlift while keeping the leg off the floor. Use a wall or chair for assistance in balancing.

# Draw the Sword/Return the Sword

## Feel it Here Back of Shoulder, Middle Back

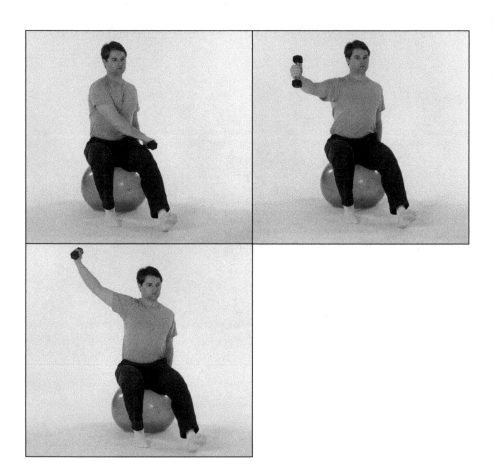

**SET-UP**

Imagine you are drawing a sword from the opposite side with a closed hand. Draw the sword across your body into an open hand position over the opposite shoulder. The motion is accomplished with the back muscles. The muscles run from the back of the shoulder through the middle back. Imagine your shoulder has a direct line of action drawn from the shoulder to the opposite hip. For an alternative, hold a light weight (shown above) in the hand that moves across the body.

# Deadlift

## Feel it Here Hips, Legs, Back

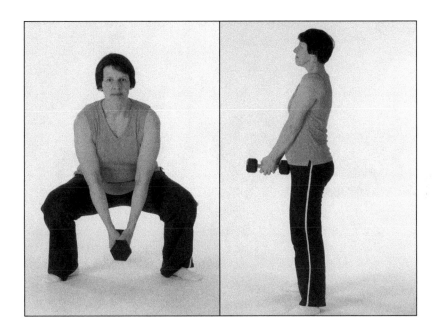

**SET-UP**

Squat with a dumbbell between your legs and perform the deadlift, slowly lifting the dumbbell up as you straighten your legs.

# Rolling Technique from Floor

## Feel it Here Core, Spine, Hips, Back

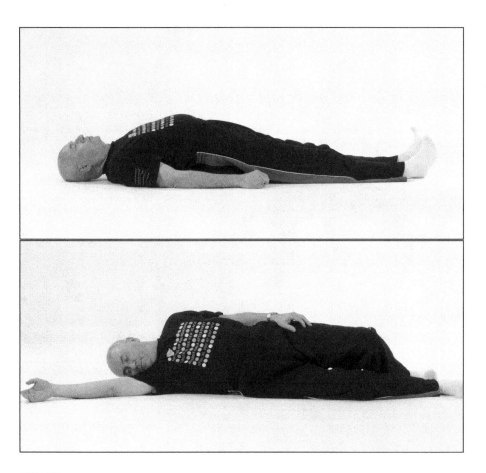

**SET-UP**

Position yourself on your back. Feel relaxed throughout your body prior to movement. Transition your body into a side-lying position by resting your head on the bottom arm. Rotate your shoulders then the spine, followed by the hips and legs. Rotating first through the spine allows you to maintain better control of your spine.

# Clock Series: Single Foot Touches

## Feel it Here Legs, Hips

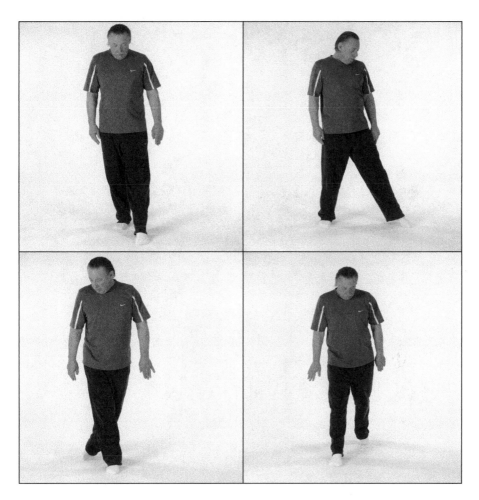

**SET-UP**

Imagine you are standing in the center of a clock face. Touch 2–3 numbers around the clock. As you become more comfortable, touch more numbers, then switch feet.

*Images should be read clockwise.*

79

# Shoulders/Torso Stretch

## Feel it Here Chest, Core, Shoulders

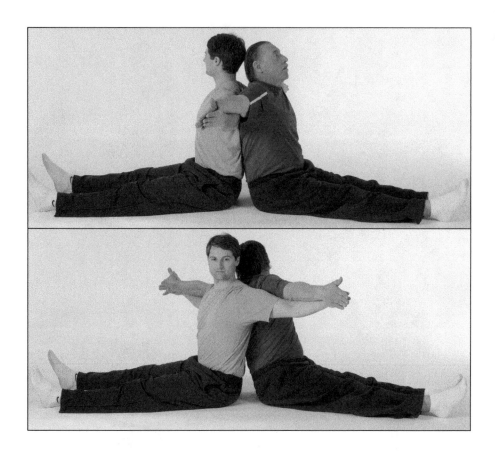

**SET-UP**

Sit back to back with your partner. Place palms in contact and rotate in unison.

# Assisted Apley Stretch

## Feel it Here Arms, Shoulders, Chest

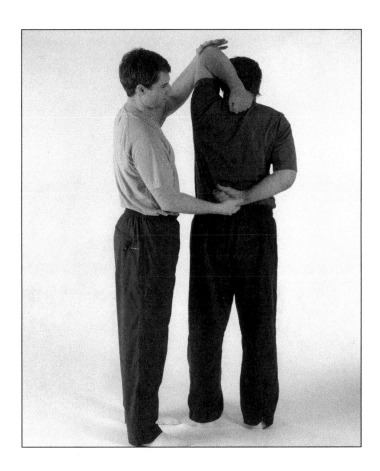

**SET-UP**

Instruct your partner to reach his or her arms over and under their shoulder blades, as shown above. Assist the elbows coming together while instructing your partner not to arch the middle back.

# Back to Back Butterfly Stretch

## Feel it Here Groin, Hips

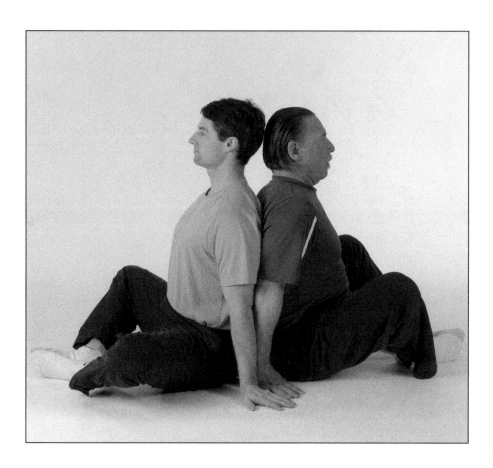

**SET-UP**

Sit back-to-back with your partner in the butterfly position, with your legs out to the side to stretch your inner thighs and hips.

# Double Hand Chest Press

**Feel it Here** Chest, Arms, Core

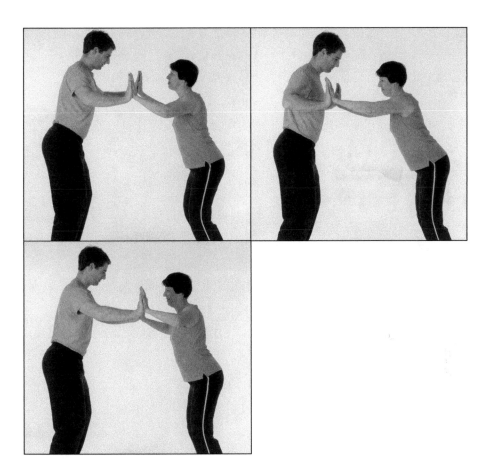

**SET-UP**

Press your palms against your partner's. Press your hands back and forth, resisting one another, but still allowing for range of motion similar to a dumbbell chest press. Be sure to stabilize backward through your core.

# Lateral Shoulder Raises

## Feel it Here Shoulders

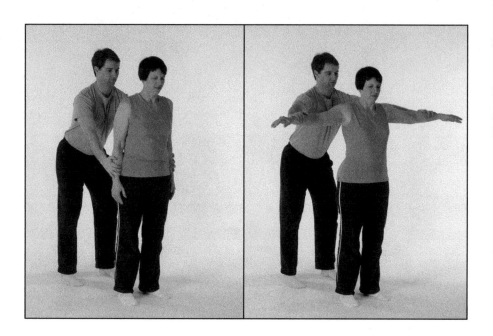

**SET-UP**

Your partner begins in a standing position. Instruct him or her to make soft fists while pushing into your resistance. Resistance is applied on the upward motion only.

# Partner Stability Pushes

## Feel it Here Core, Spine

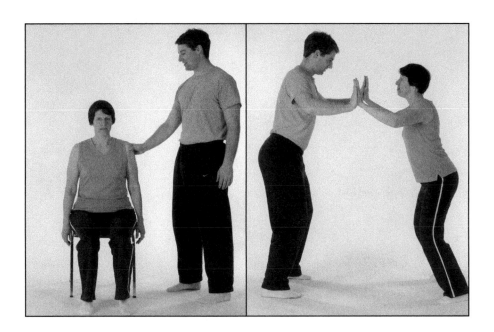

## SET-UP

Partner will start in a seated position. Instruct him or her to breathe during the entire exercise. Proceed to gently push at the shoulders, middle back, and front of the body. Once your partner feels comfortable with the seated position, try the standing position. Push your partner in the same spots.

## CHAPTER FIVE

# Exercise Programs and Progressions

How much physical activity is recommended to maintain and improve your health? The answer depends on your current level of physical activity. Are you currently active? If so, what are you doing and how often? This is very important, as the elements of any exercise program should be structured relative to your current level of activity.

Most well-rounded exercise programs should include a balance of cardiorespiratory, strength, and functional exercises.

The American College of Sports Medicine (ACSM) has developed a list of general programming recommendations that may be useful as you research what level of exercise is right for you. These are good reference points for recommended weekly activity. Keep in mind that recommendations change regularly, so it may also be helpful to research multiple resources.

## Recommendations on Quantity and Quality of Exercise

*(Source: American College of Sports Medicine)*

### Cardiorespiratory Exercise

- **Adults:** 150 minutes of moderate-intensity exercise per week.

- **Exercise recommendations:** 30-60 minutes of moderate-intensity exercise (five days per week) or 20-60 minutes of vigorous-intensity exercise (three days per week).

### Resistance Exercise

- Adults: Train major muscle groups two or three days each week.
- Two to four sets of each exercise will help adults improve strength and power.
- For each exercise, perform 8-12 repetitions to improve strength and power, 10-15 repetitions to improve strength in middle-age and older persons starting exercise, and 15-20 repetitions to improve muscular endurance.

### Functional Fitness Exercise

- **"Functional fitness training"** is recommended for two or three days per week.
- Exercises should involve motor skills (balance, agility, coordination, and gait), proprioceptive exercise training, and multifaceted activities (such as tai chi and yoga) to improve physical function and prevent falls in older adults.

In closing, getting an updated personal health history and physical assessment will provide peace of mind and sound data to measure your progress. Try to set short-term and long-term goals for yourself. For example, a short-term goal (8-12 weeks) could be to increase physical activity from 3 times to 4 times per week for a total of 120 minutes. A longer term goal (6-12 months) can include lowering blood sugars to eliminate or reduce your need for daily medication. Now is the time to start moving!

# Programs

## Introductory

**AM**
- Start the Self-Treatment and Massage progression (see page 93)
- Start the Beginner Posture Basics progression (see page 92)

**PM**
- Weekly: Complete the initial Functional Assessment and Physical Fitness Assessment (see page 91)
- Repeat the Self-Treatment and Massage progression (see page 93) or the Posture Basics progression (see page 92)

*For the Self-Treatment and Massage progression, decrease the recommended reps if you experience any fatigue or soreness.*

## Beginner Cancer Exercise Program

**AM**
- Start the Balance progression (see page 95)
- Start the Beginner Strength progression (see page 96)

**PM**
- Start the Beginner Mobility progression (see page 94)

## Intermediate

**AM**
- Start the Intermediate Strength progression (see page 97) or the Stability progression (see page 96)
- Practice the Self-Treatment and Massage progression (see page 93)
- Practice the Balance progression (see page 95)

**PM**
- Practice the Self-Treatment and Massage progression (see page 93)

## Advanced

### AM

- Practice the Balance progression (see page 95)
- Practice the Intermediate Strength progression (see page 97)

### PM

- Re-test your Physical Fitness Assessment (page 91)
- Practice the Balance progression (see page 95)

## Supplemental Program

- Practice the Posture Basics progression (see page 92)
- Start the Partner Flexibility Circuit progression (see page 98)

# Progressions

**Warm-up/Warm-down** refers to the number of minutes that should be taken to warm-up your body before a set of exercises and then the time to warm-down your body. For example, 4/4 means you take 4 minutes to warm-up and 4 minutes to warm-down.

**Rest** refers to the time taken between each set of exercises.

**RPE** refers to Rate of perceived Exertion. See page 19 for details.

## Assessments

INITIAL EVALUATION DATE (WEEK 1): _____

MID-POINT EVALUATION DATE (WEEK 8): _____

SUMMARY EVALUATION DATE (WEEK16): _____

| FUNCTIONAL ASSESSMENT | COMPLETE? (Yes/No) | DISCOMFORT? (Yes/No) | NOTE DIFFICULTY |
|---|---|---|---|
| Stair Walking | | | |
| Getting up from a Chair | | | |
| Standing with Eyes Closed | | | |
| Getting up from the Ground | | | |

| PHYSICAL FITNESS ASSESSMENT | GOAL | INITIAL | MID-POINT | SUMMARY |
|---|---|---|---|---|
| Ribs Heavy | | | | |
| Chair Sit | | | | |
| Forward Plank | | | | |
| Lateral Plank | | | | |
| Deadbug | | | | |

# Posture Basics

## Beginner Segment

**Reps:** 10 (pause 1-2 seconds at start and end of each repetition)
**Sets:** 1
**RPE:** 2-4/10

| EXERCISE | PAGE # | EQUIPMENT |
|---|---|---|
| Spinal Whip | 36 | |
| Thoracic Flex on Roller | 37 | foam roller or rolled-up towel |
| Ribcage Opener | 38 | foam roller or rolled-up towel |
| Hip Hinging | 35 | physio-ball |

## Intermediate Segment

**Reps:** 12
**Sets:** 2
**RPE:** 4/10

| EXERCISE | PAGE # | EQUIPMENT |
|---|---|---|
| Spinal Whip | 36 | |
| Alphabet T's | 39 | chair |
| Alphabet W's | 40 | chair |
| Alphabet Y's | 41 | chair |

# Self-Treatment and Massage

**Reps:** 12
**Sets:** 1
**RPE:** 4/10

| EXERCISE | PAGE # | EQUIPMENT |
|---|---|---|
| Cranial Release | 42 | foam roller or rolled-up towel |
| Glutes | 43 | foam roller or rolled-up towel |
| Sacral Release | 44 | foam roller or rolled-up towel |
| Lateral Side Bend on Physio-Ball | 45 | physio-ball, broomstick |

*Visit www.meltmethod.com for more exercises.*

# Flexibility

## Beginner Segment

**Reps:** 12
**Sets:** 2
**RPE:** 4/10

| EXERCISE | PAGE # | EQUIPMENT |
|---|---|---|
| Kneeling with Hand Across Knee | 48 | step or bench |
| Lateral Neck Stretch | 49 | chair |
| Chair Stretch | 50 | chair |
| Knee to Forehead | 51 | |

## Intermediate Segment

**Reps:** 12
**Sets:** 3
**RPE:** 6/10

| EXERCISE | PAGE # | EQUIPMENT |
| --- | --- | --- |
| Adductors with Band | 46 | theraband |
| Quads/Hip Flexors | 47 | theraband |
| Knee to Forehead | 50 | |
| Straight Leg Stretch | 52 | theraband |

# Mobility

## Beginner Segment

**Reps:** 12
**Sets:** 1-2
**RPE:** 4/10

| EXERCISE | PAGE # | EQUIPMENT |
| --- | --- | --- |
| Ankle Pumps | 53 | |
| Hip Lifters | 55 | |
| Physio-Ball Roll | 56 | physio-ball |
| Doggy Door | 60 | |

## Intermediate Segment

**Reps:** 12
**Sets:** 2
**RPE:** 4/10

| EXERCISE | PAGE # | EQUIPMENT |
|---|---|---|
| Roll and Hold | 58 | |
| Foam Roller Scissor Stretch | 59 | foam roller or rolled-up towel |
| Open Hip Squats | 54 | |
| Offering | 57 | chair |

# Balance

## Beginner Segment

**Reps/Seconds:** 10
**Sets:** 2
**RPE:** 5/10

| EXERCISE | PAGE # | EQUIPMENT |
|---|---|---|
| Standing on Toes | 66 | |
| Weight Shifting | 69 | |
| Heel to Toe Rocks | 70 | |
| Clock Series: Single Foot Touches | 79 | |

## Intermediate Segment

**Reps/Seconds:** 10
**Sets:** 2
**RPE:** 5/10

| EXERCISE | PAGE # | EQUIPMENT |
|---|---|---|
| Physio-Ball Foot Lifts | 67 | physio-ball |
| Physio-Ball Walk-Up | 68 | physio-ball |
| Heel to Toe Rocks | 70 | |

# Stability

**Reps:** 8-10
**Sets:** 3
**RPE:** 5-8/10

| EXERCISE | PAGE # | EQUIPMENT |
|---|---|---|
| Kegel | 65 | physio-ball |
| Pelvic Tilt | 61 | physio-ball |
| Chopping Movements | 62 | theraband, towel |
| Lifting Movements | 63 | theraband, towel |

# Strength

## Beginner Segment: Lower Body

**Reps:** 12
**Sets:** 2
**RPE:** 6/10

| EXERCISE | PAGE # | EQUIPMENT |
|---|---|---|
| Deadlift | 77 | dumbbell |
| Open Hip Squats | 54 | |
| Physio-Ball Walk-Up | 68 | physio-ball |
| Prone Extension Lifts | 64 | |

## Intermediate Segment: Lower Body/Core

**Reps:** 10
**Sets:** 3
**RPE:** 7/10

| EXERCISE | PAGE # | EQUIPMENT |
|---|---|---|
| Deadlift | 77 | dumbbell |
| Open Hip Squats | 54 | |
| Single Leg Deadlift | 75 | chair |
| Rolling Technique from Floor | 78 | |

## Beginner Segment: Upper Body

**Reps:** 12
**Sets:** 2
**RPE:** 6/10

| EXERCISE | PAGE # | EQUIPMENT |
|---|---|---|
| Band Rows | 72 | theraband, chair |
| Band Presses with Two Arms | 71 | theraband, chair |
| Band Pulls with One Knee Up | 73 | theraband |
| Rolling Technique from Floor | 78 | |

## Intermediate Segment: Upper Body/Core

| EXERCISE | PAGE # | EQUIPMENT |
|---|---|---|
| Rows with Triceps Extension | 74 | dumbbells |
| Band Pulls with One Knee Up | 73 | theraband |
| Draw the Sword/Return the Sword | 76 | dumbbell, physio-ball |

## Mixed Full-Body Circuit

| EXERCISE | PAGE # | EQUIPMENT |
|---|---|---|
| Deadlift | 77 | dumbbell |
| Band Pulls with One Knee Up | 73 | theraband |
| Rows with Tricep Extension * Complete two rounds of the first 3 exercises | 74 | dumbbells |
| Band Presses with Two Arms | 71 | theraband, chair |
| Open Hip Squats | 54 | |
| Single Leg Deadlift * Complete two rounds of the last 3 exercises | 75 | chair |

# Partner Flexibility Circuit

**Reps:** 12
**Sets:** 1-2
**RPE:** 5/10

| EXERCISE | PAGE # | EQUIPMENT |
|---|---|---|
| Shoulder/Torso Stretch | 80 | |
| Assisted Apley Stretch | 81 | |
| Back to Back Butterfly Stretch | 82 | |

# Partner Strength Circuit

**Reps:** 12
**Sets:** 1-2
**RPE:** 5/10

| EXERCISE | PAGE # | EQUIPMENT |
|---|---|---|
| Double Hand Chest Press | 83 | |
| Lateral Shoulder Raises | 84 | |
| Partner Stability Pushes | 85 | chair |

# RESOURCES

**American Cancer Society**
www.cancer.org

**American Institute for Cancer Research**
www.aicr.org

**Cancer.net from the American Society of Clinical Oncology (ASCO)**
www.cancer.net

**National Cancer Institute at the National Institutes of Health**
www.cancer.gov

**National Foundation for Cancer Research**
www.nfcr.org

**The University of Texas MD Anderson Cancer Center**
www.mdanderson.org

# ABOUT THE AUTHORS

**William Smith, MS, NSCA-CSCS, MEPD,** completed his B.S. in exercise science at Western Michigan University followed by a master's degree at St. John's University. While at St. John's Will was the Assistant Director of Strength and Conditioning. In addition to his many years working in fitness and medical settings, his certifications include Medical Exercise Program Director and STAR provider through Oncology Rehab Partners. Will currently teaches at UMDNJ Physical Therapy at Rutgers University.

**Jo Brielyn** is a freelance writer and author. She is a contributing writer for Hatherleigh Press and has published works in several print and online publications. Jo also owns and maintains the Creative Kids Ideas (www.creative-kidsideas.com) and Good for Your Health (www.good-for-yourhealth.com) websites. For more information about Jo's upcoming projects or to contact her, visit www.JoBrielyn.com. Jo resides in Central Florida with her husband and two daughters.

**Kenneth Adler, M.D.** is an Assistant Clinical Professor of Medicine at the New Jersey Medical School and Associate Member of the Cancer Institute of New Jersey. After receiving his medical education at Albany Medical College of Union University, Dr. Adler went on to specialize in Hematology-Oncology, and currently serves as Attending Physician in Hematology-Oncology at the Carol Simon Cancer Center in Morristown, New Jersey. He is a Fellow of the American College of Physicians, The Oncology Society of New Jersey, The American Society of Hematology, and the American Society of Clinical Oncology. He is currently Chairman of the New Jersey Commission on Cancer Research, and a member of Regional Cancer Care Associates.

# Also in the *Exercises for* Series...

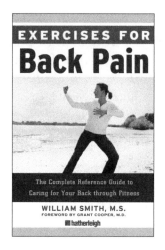

*Exercises for Back Pain*
ISBN 978-1-57826-304-2

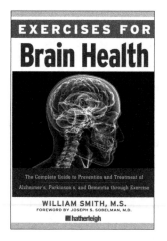

*Exercises for Brain Health*
ISBN 978-1-57826-316-5

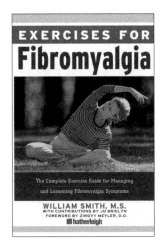

*Exercises for Fibromyalgia*
ISBN 978-1-57826-361-5

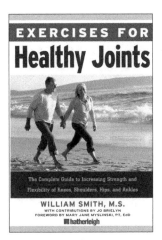

*Exercises for Healthy Joints*
ISBN 978-1-57826-344-8

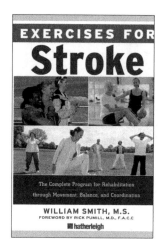

*Exercises for Stroke*
ISBN 978-1578263172

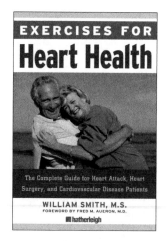

*Exercises for Heart Health*
ISBN 978-1578263035